RED LIGHT TH

A Comprehensive Guide to Red Light Treatment

COPYRIGHT

All rights reserved. This book may not be reproduced, transmitted by any means without the explicit permission of the copyright owner.

MAC ANDREWS © 2020

Table of Content

TABLE OF CONTENT 1

INTRODUCTION 2

Medical Disclaimer 3

A Beginner's Guide 4

History of Red Light Therapy 5

How Does Red Light Therapy (RLT) Work? 7

Scientific Proof that RLT Works 13

Red Light Therapy at Home 38

Important Considerations before Choosing an ELT Device
.... 39

Red Light Therapy Dosage or Photobiomodulation 46

Tips for Red Light Therapy 51

Risk, Side Effects, and Contraindications 59

Conclusion 63

Introduction

Red Light Therapy or treatment, also known as bio-stimulation, lightbox therapy, Photobiomodulation, or low-level light therapy (LLLT) has become very popular. Since this therapy can be considered "alternative", many swear by it. They are using it to improve wellbeing, reduce wrinkles and minimize the impact of aging, improve recovery after surgery, and for many other personal needs. However, this includes but is not limited to easing sore muscles, enhancing hair growth, moisturizing dry skin, improving weight loss, and helping with winter depression.

This complete guidebook on Red Light Therapy will gaze into all there is to know about Red Light Therapy. In this guidebook, we shall:

- Nurture an in-depth understanding of the concept of Red Light Therapy;
- Find out if it works and also discover how it works;

- Examine the many benefits of using this alternative therapy, especially if you intend to use it to enhance personal wellbeing;

Medical Disclaimer

The content of this book is strictly for informational purposes and does not take the place of professional medical advice, treatment, or diagnosis. Seek professional guidance and advice from your health care provider if you have questions on any serious medical condition.

A Beginner's Guide

Red light therapy or treatment can be seen as an alternative yet heliotherapy therapy or treatment that exposes the skin to near-infrared light and red light at very precise wavelengths (630 to 880) to treat skin-related problems like wounds, wrinkles, and scars, as well as enhance overall cellular and personal health and wellbeing.

The science and reasoning behind the use of Red Light Therapy date back to the millennia. Hence, to thoroughly understand Red Light Therapy, we have to know how humankind has been using both natural and artificial light for different means and ends, including as a treatment option.

History of Red Light Therapy

Red Light Therapy is a form of heliotherapy, which is a type of therapy that exposes the skin to light at precise wavelengths. This type of light therapy has been in use for thousands of years, possibly since modern civilization began.

For instance:

Historical researchers believe that some residents of Ancient Rome, Athens, and Egypt used light therapy in various forms. An example is making use of the sun's light to improve people's overall wellbeing. The Ancient Indians in 1500 BCE were using their knowledge of herbs with light from the sun to treat several skin problems like scabs and wounds.

Phototherapy in modern times should be grateful to the physician from Faroese known as Neil Finsen. He is believed to be the first human to develop an artificial source of light that can specifically use light to heal. He demonstrated this by using light to treat various skin infections including lupus vulgaris.

According to Wikipedia, Finsel designed red lights around the late 1800s to early 1900s. Then he used these lights to treat lesions that were caused by smallpox. In 1903, the received the Nobel Prize in Medicine.

Heliotherapy has since the early 1900s seen great advances. It has also been used for many means like using red lights created especially for food production. A technology like this was used by NASA in the 1990s to cultivate food in space. The red light was also used for healing as was used in RLT as well as other forms of heliotherapies like LED light treatment.

Many heliotherapies are quite particular about the nature and amount of exposure, which is the wavelength of light and time of exposure to the light. This is because most of the modern therapies that fall under the heliotherapy classification make use of specialized light technologies like lasers, LED light, full-spectrum lights, dichroic lamps, or polychromatic polarize lights. Since the use of these specialized lights is safe on the skin, over-exposure to some of them can sometimes damage the skin or area of treatment. This can necessitate some caution.

How Does Red Light Therapy (RLT) Work?

According to Dictionary.com, the electromagnetic spectrum is "the range or number of frequencies or wavelengths electromagnetic radiation can extend." This is the reason it is so important:

A session of red light therapy is supposed to expose a certain amount of skin to a certain red light wavelength for a certain amount of time, which often falls between 10 to 60 minutes. The light, through this exposure, penetrates the skin and interacts with the cell nuclei, which then offers some therapeutic benefits.

Red light is seen as a major part of the electromagnetic spectrum which consists of seven electromagnetic waves. They are Gamma Rays, X-Rays, Ultraviolet Waves, Visible Light Rays, Infrared Waves, Microwaves, and Radio Waves.

Red light, along with other color hues namely orange, yellow, green, blue, indigo, and violet, falls under this spectrum. Hence, this light can be seen by the naked eye. Each color in this large visible light rays classification has a particular frequency or wavelength. These frequencies are measured using nanometers (nm). These rays possess a wavelength range of 400 to 880 nm.

The ability of the light to penetrate the skin is determined by the frequency length, this means that the longer the wavelength, the deeper the penetration. Many red lights have a capacity of about 630 to 880 nm, which gives them the ability to penetrate as deeply as 5-10 millimeters into the skin. This means that light can reach all the layers of the skin.

The integumentary system, which has its largest organ as the skin, is a vital bodily system that serves as a protective barrier against viruses or diseases. This helps the human body to retain its fluids, remove bodily waste, and regulate body temperature. By implication, the skin has billions of cells.

Cells are also powerhouses that drive you. They have mitochondria in them which are billions of cell stations that your body utilizes to generate energy on a cellular level. To enjoy excellent cellular health, one important molecule to have is the adenosine triphosphate (ATP). Our cells would likely starve without it. More so, if there is no energy required for cellular metabolism (including internal and external functions of the body requiring energy like walking, healing, digestion, repair, breathing, etc.), they just might die off, and we would too.

When a red light of therapeutic grade is shone on the skin, it affects the mitochondria's functionalities by activating the production of additional ATP. This is because light can penetrate the skin very deep and come in contact with cells in their billions.

As soon as red light activates higher ATP production, the biochemical effect resulting from this will enhance both cellular and mitochondrial functionality (efficient production of energy). The higher ATP production will cause the cells to easily access the energy they require for optimal repairs, rejuvenation, and function.

To better understand the effect of red light therapy on cells and ATP production, you should understand that all cells require natural light to power the processes that generate the energy your body uses every day. It does this without shining any special red light on your skin and cells. If there is no red light therapy, your cells will still power this process with the natural red light.

Red light therapy is meant to control the times when your skin is exposed to the red light's healing spectrum. Additionally, it is to shine a particular wavelength of light directly on the skin to enhance cellular activity by activating an ATP production process that is leaner and very efficient.

The science behind this procedure believes that the body creates ATP in two ways: aerobic and anaerobic. Oxygen is required for anaerobic, while no oxygen is called aerobic. This happens in a process called cellular respiration. This process involves the body using various means like food, water, and the air we breathe to generate the energy we require for optimal survival and operation. Aerobic ATP generation is the most effective of the two processes, and since it produces most of the energy, the body prefers using it to create ATP and energy.

The generation of aerobic ATP is in four primary stages; the first stage is glycolysis while the second stage is pyruvate oxidation. In the glycolysis stage, our body will use all available resources (air, food, and water) to synthesize the pyruvates. In the pyruvate oxidation stage, the body will oxidize the pyruvate into Acetyl CoA. The production process of Acetyl CoA results in the generation of CO_2 compounds which turn to aerobic energy that 95% of the cells in the body use.

The citric acid cycle makes up the third stage, while oxidative phosphorylation is the fourth stage. The citric acid cycle stage stands as the primary objective. This stage involves giving the body Acetyl CoA which was made in the second stage. It is then oxidized and used in creating coenzymes namely NADH and FADHs. In the oxidative phosphorylation stage, NADH and

FADHs, which are coenzymes, are conducted by electrons into an electron transport chain, thereby creating energy.

The routine use of a red light machine as prescribed will ensure that the nitric oxide that the ATP creation process made does not get too oxidative and harmful to cells. When mitochondria are stimulated to create more ATP, cells tend to function better, heal faster, repair faster, as well as fight ailments, viruses, and so on.

Additionally, if you expose the skin to near-infrared lights and therapeutic red light at certain wavelengths, you are promoting better cellular signaling and communication. When these cells communicate better, there will be an improved synthesis of protein, enhanced cell functionality, and activity of the enzymes.

Due to the way red and NIL lights affect nitric oxide production within the cells, they help in enhancing antioxidants production. Antioxidants help to protect the cells from chronic and oxidative stress and mutations that are capable of impairing cell health, circulation, and many other vital bodily functions with the inclusion of people connected with general health and overall wellbeing.

Exposure to either red light or near-infrared wavelengths is not harmful unlike exposure to microwaves, ultraviolet waves, and higher gamma rays' spectrums. This is as a result of the treatment being done in a controlled environment like a medical center or licensed spa or using a high-grade red light device in your home. Hence, there is very little chance that the light wavelengths that were generated by pure red light would burn the skin. This is what makes the use of red light therapy a safe option for many people.

Take note that to be safe, do not use red light therapy or any other light therapy without consulting a health professional. A professional will make sure your treatment sessions are done in a regulated and safe environment.

In the next section, we will be looking at the many benefits of both red light therapy and heliotherapy as proven by science.

Scientific Proof that RLT Works

It has been shown and proven through scientific research that RLT works and has many benefits.

As seen in previous sections, RLT works through a process of shining a penetrating red on the skin, which is a therapeutic light meant to stimulate cellular production of ATP. The ATP is the molecule that ensures that resources are transmuted into the cellular energy which our bodies need and use for powering many metabolic processes including the ones related to healing of cells and rejuvenation.

Several research studies show that safe and consistent exposure to red light therapy can result in biochemical processes which may have the following benefits:

RLT improves sleep

Better sleep implies better rest and requires more energy and productivity during the day. So far, red light therapy has been effective in improving sleep patterns by normalizing and enhancing circadian rhythms as well as the ability of the cell to produce melatonin. Melatonin is the hormone that is produced primarily to help control the sleep-and-wake the upcycle of your body.

Morita, T. and Tokura, H. researched to determine the effect of daytime red light therapy sessions on the ability of the body to produce melatonin. It was determined that daytime exposure to pure red light led to increasing in the production of melatonin as well as a rationalized circadian rhythm. This congruency means that red light therapy sessions in the day time will result in better sleep and rest.

How it works

Poor sleep patterns have negative consequences and effects both short and long-term. For instance, poor sleep patterns affect our hormonal balance, which in turn affects our mood and wellbeing. These patterns also cause low energy, subsequently decreasing output and productivity and causing a lot of negative consequences like inability to attain set goals.

Also, a feeling of chronic tiredness can cause mental health complications like stress, depression, and anxiety, as well as attendant conditions like rapid weight loss or gain, insulin imbalances that make it hard for the body to know when it requires sustenance, and increased risk of having type 2 diabetes.

Some studies have gone as far as concluding that poor sleep can cause reduced cognitive function like decreased mental clarity and low attention span.

It was important to outline how abnormal sleep patterns can reduce your wellbeing overall percentage because it made a background that will assist you in understanding how red light therapy can make sure you sleep better.

First note that our sleep cycles are dependent on light, i.e. light is a determinant factor of how your body chooses when it needs sleep. The body uses manmade and natural light to choose when to produce the hormones necessary for the body to have a circadian system or rhythm that is operationally effective.

Since our modern lives are so full of artificial lights like bulbs and screens, it can result in a confused circadian pattern, which throws your cycle of sleep off balance. This can make it harder for you to rest well, fall asleep naturally, and wake up feeling rejuvenated and refreshed.

Secondly, some lights harm our circadian rhythm as well as our sleeping and resting. To be more specific, we shall dwell on blue light.

It is quite common to be exposed to blue light in the form of screens like televisions, laptops, monitors, phones, tablets, and so on. Since most people are now used to being exposed to blue light especially in the evening and at night, our bodies have adjusted to this and interpret it to mean it should stay awake because of the light outside.

Several clinical studies have shown that sessions of red light therapy held in the evening can improve sleep patterns. Since pure red light has a lower temperature, exposing your body to such light wavelength in the evening will tell your body that the temperature of the light has changed to a low one (evening or night) and that it is time for it to prepare to rest by producing the melatonin hormone.

Taiwanese researchers in 2013 tried to determine the electroencephalography EEG (state of brain activity) before, during and after the sessions of red light therapy sessions. This was done by analyzing each of the study participants' EEGs. In their conclusion, exposure to a pure, therapeutic red light in the evening or night was very effective in combating common sleep disorders.

As we saw earlier, one of the reasons red light therapy is so effective in "alternative sleep therapy" is because of its effect on the signals that trigger melatonin production. Since pure grade red light and near-infrared light have low temperatures, exposing your body to them during the daytime can have a seriously positive effect on natural melatonin production.

We can conclude logically from the different research studies discussed here that red light therapy is very effective as an alternative form of sleep therapy, to the extent that lying in pure red light at evening time can make you fall asleep easily and even sleep better.

In research on how red light therapy improves sleep, Margaret N. and Michael H. showed that patients who suffered from traumatic brain injury and who were subjected to 1-hour, red light therapy sessions carried out 18 times, slept one hour longer than others and awoke to feel well-rested and refreshed.

RLT Benefits for the Skin

Different studies have concluded that when the safe red light is used in a controlled environment, it offers many benefits for the skin.

RLT therapy has been known to enhance the skin's overall health. As seen earlier, the impact of red light on the skin cells at the point where ATP production is stimulated helps to enhance production, leading to overall cellular wellbeing. This, in turn, means the skin will be smoother, healthier, and acne-free, collagen production will be boosted which results in wrinkle-free skin. Enhanced cell health will lead to less scarring of the skin and a faster ability to heal.

There are a lot of estheticians, dermatologists, professionals, celebrities, and trustworthy publications like CNN who have publicly acknowledged that red light therapy has positive effects on the skin.

How it works

The core of red light therapy is shining a wavelength of red light that is controlled. Due to this controlled red light therapy of 660-850 nm wavelengths, your skin will be safe when exposed to these wavelengths of light. This happens because even if the red light is not shone on the cells, they can still absorb these wavelengths of light from the environment and use it for powering cellular functionality.

When you are in charge of how your cells receive pure red light wavelength which they need to function effectively, the result is a controlled stimulation of ATP production which leads to improved skin functionality.

Better functioning skin cells along with cells that circulate well in different skin layers and Electron

Transport Chain, often result in lower oxidation. Lower oxidation, by interpretation, is an efficient process of cellular energy production, functionality, better circulation, better protection from the sun's harmful rays, reduced skin inflammation, and overall better skin health and appearance.

Maria Emilia de Abreu Chaves et al. conducted a research study on increasing the circulation of cells within the different skin layers. It was noted during this research that when red light therapy is used continually in a controlled way, there is an increase in circulation by ensuring the effective functioning of the cells and the tissues get the energy, oxygen support, and nutrition they require to function properly.

Also, the process reduces the oxidative stress on cells thereby enhancing the ability of the skin to detoxify itself—meaning there is a lesser need for products and 'skin detoxes'—and heal scar tissues and wounds faster and better.

RLT offers a lot of benefits to the skin.

For example:

The anti-inflammatory part: When a therapeutic-grade red light is shone on your skin, a biochemical process is stimulated and this enhances the ability of your skin cells to generate energy for themselves as well as for the overall layer of the skin and other body parts. Since our organs are interconnected in a web, the cells on the skin will heal and rejuvenate better and faster to cause a healing effect. This effect can be passed onto other parts of the body.

An aspect of the red light therapy's healing effect on the skin cells is that it helps to reduce inflammation and stress. When a therapeutic grade red light is again shone on the skin cells, their functionality is enhanced. This means that your cells can get better energy, oxygen flow, and blood, which means the skin will heal, repair, and rejuvenate better.

More specifically, Dr. Michael Hamblin in a research study noted that "skin cells consider the wavelengths used for the red light and near-infrared light therapy a form of mild stress. When you expose these skin cells to this form of mild stress, it activates their need to self-protect (and to protect you too). When the cells are in the self-protect mode, they function more efficiently and are very adept at creating the antioxidants they need to fight any inflammatory effect caused by the mild stress."

As seen in a study that was published in Medical Science, red light therapy is very effective in reducing inflammation because RLT treatment has a therapeutic effect on post-surgery inflammation. Post-surgery inflammation, when reduced, could lead to more pain relief, less irritation, and less wound swelling. Due to improved cell functionality, faster healing and recovery time, which implies with consultation, it can be very beneficial to use red light therapy after a session of surgery because of wound management, which also stimulates the cells to work better and heal faster.

Lee, J.H., et al. in an oral study said that when red light therapy is used on the mouth, that is when the periodontal cells are exposed to therapeutic red light, inflammation could reduce and the ability of the cells to stave off mouth toxins like E. coli and P. gingivalis will be enhanced.

Also, red light therapy affects muscle soreness or musculoskeletal soreness.

In a research study that was published in 2008, it was noted that when heliotherapy is controlled, it reduces the symptoms of muscle soreness significantly. Researchers in another study from Brazil revealed that the use of red light therapy machine before exercise led to a high level of reduction of muscle soreness/inflammation and post-workout pain.

RLT Benefits for Weight Loss

Firstly, eating healthy and consistently engaging in physical activity like exercise remain the best way to lose weight. There are many ways to improve fat loss and weight. There is intermittent fasting, taking supplements like garcinia Cambogia for weight loss, and detoxing for instance. RLT can be effectively used as an alternative strategy for weight loss coupled with healthy eating and adequate workout. RLT can be used to improve the ability of the body to burn fat.

Different studies have shown how red light therapy can influence weight loss, weight gain, or retainment positively. Researchers, in particular, have noted the effectiveness of red light therapy as an alternative weight loss strategy due to how its effects act on the adipocytes cells (the cells responsible for storing fat in your body).

Borghi-Silva A, Paolillo F.R., et al. in 2011, published a studied that revealed what was discovered by the researchers after subjecting women aged 25 to 55 years as study participants to both treadmill workouts and red light therapy. In the study, participants were categorized into two: women who only engaged in treadmill exercises, and those who engaged in treadmill exercises and 2 red light therapy sessions every week. The study-measure was to determine the influence of red light therapy on cellulite.

These researchers showed the remarkable differences between both study groups. The starkest difference was that the second group comprising those that engaged in treadmill exercises and 2 sessions of red light therapy every week showed remarkable enhancement of thigh cellulite. It was then concluded by these researchers that engaging in both exercise and RLT leads to an aesthetically pleasing body as well as the increased loss of fat.

The International Journal of Endocrinology (the study of hormones and glands in medicine) in 2012 published a study in which researchers came to the conclusion that light influences eating patterns, which can also influence levels of hunger and satiety.

They concluded that whenever the hormones and signals of your hunger and satiety are not functioning properly, it results in reduced ability to regular when to eat and when not to eat. This reduced ability can result in conditions like binge eating, as well as several hormone-regulations conditions like type 2 diabetes and cellular attached to fat storage in lipid form. Near-infrared light and red light therapy help to increase cellular activity, which in effect means that while the cells work better, there is also increased capacity to release fat lipids. Red light therapy together with healthy eating and regular exercise can make you lose weight dramatically.

How it works

Red light therapy is a very effective alternative form of weight loss therapy because it activates better adipocyte (fat in the body that regulate cells) activity. As soon as red and near-infrared lights make contact with the skin, a biochemical reaction occurs which triggers improved activity in the fat cells that will make the cells to release lipids they may be carrying when they are activated.

Additionally, researchers have concluded that RLT is effective as an alternative weight-loss management system because it can regulate the production of many hunger hormones, especially ghrelin and leptin.

Several research findings are in support of red light therapy as an alternative weight loss strategy or system which, together with eating healthy and exercising adequately, can have benefits in increased metabolism and fat loss.

If you want to lose weight, it may be because you want to sculpt the 'body of your dreams'. Hence, you may choose any therapy at your disposal like targeted surgeries and body sculpting techniques.

It has been scientifically proven that the use of RLT for weight loss along with other good-health strategies can go a long way to increase your chances of losing so much fat and help contour your body so that you will have the body you desire.

One of the effective ways of contouring the body is by using handheld RLT devices because they will let you understand how to target and maneuver better. When you allow for improved targeting of particular 'fatty' areas like love handles, underarms, and thighs, red light therapy ensures far better and targeted cellular stimulation of the fat cells mentioned earlier. When you use pure red light to cause increased activity in places that may carry fat, your body may release these lipids in cells, which eases the weight loss process.

In a study conducted after a double-blind study in 2011 with results that were published in the Journal of Obesity Surgery, the researchers have concluded that red light therapy may lead to slimming the waistline. In the study, participants were allowed to access sessions of red light therapy of 635 to 80nm for four weeks. The focus of the researchers was on the effect of these therapy sessions on the waistline girth. It was concluded in their study that exposure to red light at 635-80nm wavelengths will make for a great waistline sculpting tool.

Many other studies are in support of the findings in the above-mentioned study. A study like this appears in Lasers in Surgery Medicine. Researchers in this research study tried finding out the effectiveness of using RLT as a targeted weight loss tool-its effectiveness in helping a person lose weight in targeted areas. After participants were offered sessions of red light and near-infrared light therapy, the researchers discovered that these resulted in a massive loss of body fat in important areas like the underarms, thighs, etc.

In 2013, another study published that researchers found that exposure to pure red light at a wavelength of 635 nm resulted in contoured hips and thighs. Some of the study's participants experienced a reduction of not less than 2.99 inches of their bigger body size.

Researchers in a recent study in 2018 tried determining the exact effect of red light therapy on the loss of body fat most especially in endurance training. The research concluded after the study showed that participants who had sessions of red light therapy pre-exercise had better synthesis and loss of body fat compared to the placebo. This means that their bodies were able to burn fat quicker during sessions of endurance training and long afterward.

Red light and infrared light therapy are also very effective as a tool for obesity management. Brazilian researchers assessed the results of these research findings which offered red light therapy of 64 obese women from 20-40 years and concluded that when this therapy is coupled with exercise, there will be a potential to cause greater weight loss. According to the researchers, "when obese women engage in light therapy and exercise, in addition to increased weight loss, they displayed significant metabolic flexibility."

There are a lot of research findings supporting the use of red light therapy to lose weight or fat if you search well for it. As a red light therapy alternative, weight loss therapy offers more control and targeting, and it can be done safely at home.

The marketplace has so much to offer in terms of being effective, usable at home or handheld red and near-infrared lights that can be used whenever you wish – keeping the guidelines recommended by your physician in mind – and the ones that can be used for targeting particular problem areas like love handles.

Since pure red light is quite safe and has many research findings supporting its effectiveness as a tool for weight management, provided your physician had been consulted, nothing is hindering red light therapy being used as a body-sculpting and weight loss tool.

RLT Benefits for Enhancing Muscle Recovery and Performance

So far, it is quite easy to see the positive effects red light therapy has on performance and muscle recovery.

Firstly, when the pure red light is exposed to different layers of the skin, there is an increase in cellular metabolism. How does this help performance and muscle recovery?

When these red light therapy sessions are undertaken, the cells are activated into producing additional ATP/energy, there is an increase in cell activity, and the access of the cells to cleaner, efficient energy will increase the performance and make them function more effectively.

More so, engaging in red light therapy can positively affect cellular performance as well as the overall performance of the body and brain since it stimulates cells in a manner that results in better cellular communication and circulation.

How it works

Top athletes and professionals have been known to advocate for red light therapy in increasing physical performance, growing muscles, and speeding up recovery after the training. So far, many research studies have shown how effective RLT is as a tool for performance and recovery, this is why NBA teams, NFL all-professionals, professional gyms, and boxers now use it.

A study in 2011, researchers were out to determine how red light and near-infrared light therapy affected strength training in men. They noted that combining strength training with light therapy results in better muscular performance and recovery, especially when it is compared to results that are displayed by a test group.

In a controlled study in 2014, researchers observed that red light therapy can increase their grip strength. Research in this particular study noted that there was a 52% increase in hand-based or grip exercises in the course of strength training sessions.

Researchers in a scientific trial that was conducted in 2016 tried to determine the effect that red light therapy sessions would have on strength training in 18-35-year-old men. It was concluded that men engaged in strength training and sessions of red light therapy increased torque/mobility as they were engaging in exercises that were leg-based like leg extensions and presses. These researchers noted that when a person engages in phototherapy before sessions of strength training the result is enhanced strength which is very beneficial for post-exercise recovery.

Tons of research studies have proven the effectiveness of RLT in enhancing endurance. With better endurance, you can exercise for longer despite the type of exercise you are carrying out.

In another example, a controlled trial in 2018 wanted to know the influence of red light therapy on endurance in both healthy men and women. The treadmill was their preferred exercise machine. It was concluded that "engaging in light therapy before exercise increases oxygen uptake, increase how long volunteers could exercise before hitting the point of exhaustion, and significantly improves fat loss." The researchers proposed that carrying out red light therapy before engaging in endurance training can significantly increase endurance by more than 2 times.

Brazilian researchers in 2018 and futsal players came together to do a triple-blind study. Firstly, Futsal is a popular Brazilian indoor soccer that is not like soccer. The game is quite challenging and demands more endurance because of the smaller playing field.

After pro-Futsal players had been allowed to access sessions of red light therapy before matches, then analyzing their findings, the researchers decided that participants in the red light therapy may out-endure this placebo group. In their conclusion, "Red light therapy significantly improved how long a player could stay on the pitch and had an overall positive effect on the various biochemical markers segregated for monitoring pre-exercise."

The results of the Futsal study mentioned above were backed by two trial studies that were conducted by the same team. In one of such studies, researchers want to determine if red light therapy has any effect on a professional cyclist's performance. Researchers in this study concluded that engaging in sessions of red light therapy before bouts of professional cycling increased the time it took for one pro-cyclist to get exhausted.

Researchers in the second research study were bent on determining the VO2 kinetics in the course of cycling test (the rate at which a body responds to an increase in oxygen demand during workouts). The study came up with similar results – RLT pre-cycling tests can increase exhaustion time as well as oxygen uptake.

Many research studies concluded that another way through which red light therapy enhances performance and muscle recovery is through enhancing speed – which is particular to running.

Researchers in 2016 studied the key markers for assessing physical performance in pro-rugby players. At the end of their research study, their findings were presented to illustrate red light therapy effectiveness. They proved that, in rugby players, RLT results in faster running, better sprint times, and improved muscle recovery.

Brazilian researchers in 2018 conducted another study in which they wanted to know if sessions of red light therapy before running exercises would result in efficient and faster running. The double-blind study had three groups: a placebo, a control group that did not get a session of red light therapy, and men who got these treatments.

From the results of the research, it was shown that the men who took place in red light therapy were the best performers: they ran faster, ran longer, and their peal velocities were higher compared to those in the other 2 groups.

Many research studies show that red light therapy is very effective as a tool for muscle growth or enhancement.

In 2010, one of such studies which were conducted by Kelencz CA, Munoz IS, etc. and published in Photomedicine and Laser Surgery, the researchers tried using both genders to know whether red light therapy causes less exhaustion and more muscles. They concluded that the group that took part in the red light therapy showed significant increases in both muscular activity and muscular strength.

In The American Journal of Physical Medicine and Rehabilitation, a published research study showed that RLT and near-infrared light therapies could lead to the size and bulk of muscles. This is done by promoting the cellular growth of muscle hypertrophy and healthy muscle tissues.

In a unique study that was published in the European Journal of Applied Physiology made use of two groups – a placebo/control group, and a group that underwent red light therapy –to determine the growth in muscle and strength, as well as the differences between both groups. In their conclusion, they noted that the muscle of the group coupling exercise with red light therapy was stronger and thicker (by not less than 50%).

With all, we know concerning near-infrared light therapy and therapy with red light, it is clear that red light therapy will work great for muscular recovery, performance, and strength. With an increase in cellular activity, which happens when the human body or skin is exposed to a pure red light or infrared light at the correct wavelengths, there is a decrease in inflammation while there is an increase in other cellular functionalities.

More so, due to its anti-oxidation effect on cells, there is a reduction in muscle fatigue which then leads to enhanced performance and increase in heat hormone production, which are vital proteins that ensure the cell is healthy and operates well by safeguarding them against chronic oxidation, mutations, then decay, and subsequent death.

Also, light therapy causes enhanced blood flow. When your muscles get more blood, they work better, endure more, and rejuvenate faster.

RLT Benefits for Improved Joint Pain Inflammation

The body often makes use of natural light and pure red light to increase the activity in the lymphatic system, toxins management system, and the body's waste. It has been shown by scientific research that increased activity in this system minimizes swelling and inflammation.

This means that due to this effect against inflammation and pain, the use of red light therapy for ailments like arthritis that are inflammation-based can be very helpful. As shown by many research studies, red light therapy is very effective since it acts on cell nuclei, and by so doing, it treats the root cause of the issue.

In a photomedicine research study conducted by Brazilian researchers in 2018, it was concluded that a significant reduction in cytokine after undergoing red light therapy. According to their research, red light therapy can speed up an inflammatory response by stimulating the regeneration of cells. RLT helps to activate the ability of the cells to create ATP, which is the most significant molecule.

Several studies have shown that RLT is safe and effective for joint pain management and managing arthritis.

For example:

Effects of RLT on Osteoarthritis: Several studies have tried to determine if photomedicine is effective in managing Osteoarthritis and knee pain.

Since the red light device is very effective in activating cellular metabolism, it is only natural that the red light therapy would effectively manage pains that are knee-related. In two different Brazilian studies that were conducted in 2018, it was concluded that combining light stretching and exercising with red light therapy was very effective at treating osteoarthritis.

It was specifically noted by one of the teams that, "after red light therapy and stretching or exercise, study participants illustrated significantly reduced levels of knee pain and increased mobility after 90 days of light stretching."

As far as pain management is concerned, researchers have proven that RLT is a very effective tool for general pain management. An Australian Journal of Physiotherapy review team reviewed 11 clinical trials on photomedicine and red light therapy and concluded that all participants across the clinical trials displayed a remarkable decrease in joint pains, including general knee pain.

Also, RLT has proven to be very effective at managing different forms of joint pains, including hand and wrist pains. In a review study that was published by Paolillo AR, Paolillo FR, et al. in the Lasers in Medical Science, it was concluded that light therapy is effective at treating hand osteoarthritis (hand pain) in women, and most of these women reported substantial reductions in increased mobility and pain.

Baltzer AW, Ostapczuk MS, Stosch D. in 2016 wanted to know if low-level laser therapy (red light therapy) has positive effects on Bouchard's osteoarthritis (a bony outgrowth) and Heberden's osteoarthritis (a swelling condition). There were 34 participants in the study. According to the research team, red light therapy has resulted in significant improvements in reduced swelling, hand mobility, and positive effects on the size of the ring.

Lots of other studies support the use of red light therapy as a great way of managing spine pains that are caused by many conditions like ankylosing spondylitis. In one of such studies published in 2016, researchers observed that participants who used red light therapy with stretching displayed enhanced mobility and substantial reductions in spinal pain.

It can be concluded from the many research studies discussed here that many research findings have proven that red light therapy is very effective and beneficial in so many ways.

Because red light therapy is drug-free and non-invasive, it can be safely used in most people, and they are contraindications. More so, because red light therapy is controlled, especially in terms of light wavelength used during therapy, it has not shown any long-term negative side-effects.

Also, it can be inferred that red light therapy or popularity has seen substantial growth as the technology is advancing. There are now handheld RLT devices and lots of treatment centers around the globe, so anyone can make use of this alternative therapy.

Since red light therapy treatment centers now have different procedures and regulations, we will concentrate more on using red light therapy at home and deconcentrating treatments within these centers.

Red Light Therapy at Home

Since light therapy (or photobiomodulation) has significantly advanced, there are a lot of options for red light therapy at our disposal. As noted earlier, this kind of treatment can be received at alternative therapies clinics or professional spas.

As an example, you may seek professional heliotherapy treatments from a local beauty salon which may have a professional red light device or modified tanning bed that will allow for full-body treatments. Many of these devices are often too costly for regular home users. A session of red light therapy in most of these establishments costs $25 to $100 per session.

It was earlier mentioned that as a result of technological advancements, especially the advancements in photobiomodulation, red light therapy can be safely used at home and home-based red light devices are more popular compared to in-clinic therapy sessions or treatments.

After you might have consulted your physician and chosen to begin using red light therapy at home, the major challenge you may encounter is that of choice. This is because there are plenty of at-home red light treatments available.

Choosing a red light device that suits you requires that you keep in mind a couple of things.

Important Considerations before Choosing an ELT Device

Having fully understood the concept of how red light therapy works, you may want to start using it to maximize all the benefits. Hence, the need to buy an RLT device.

You may want to consider the following important considerations before making a purchase:

1. Device's wavelength and intensity

The wavelength of an RLT device cannot be overlooked when purchasing and it is important to use the right wavelength of red light.

Most of these at-home red light therapy devices come with a wavelength of 630 to 700nm. If your dermatologist or health professional advised its use, you could also look for devices with a wavelength of 600nm as the light from that device is more orange than red. Devices of a higher wavelength of 800 to 900nm are called near-infrared.

When choosing an RLT device with the right wavelength, consider going for those in the mid-600-low/mid800nm range; devices that fall within this wavelength often have the most impact on the process of ATP generation.

Tip: When researching on which device would be best for you, concentrate on getting a device with a wavelength of 660nm-850nm since they can better impact on cells the most.

In red light therapy, it is the intensity that defines the amount of energy that a device delivers to the cells. The best thing to do here is to go with devices that can deliver 4-6 Joules/cm2 of the body's cells. Devices that can be this intense are the most effective as proven by many research studies, including the ones that are supported by NASA. Devices with higher intensity are more effective for conditions like inflammation and joint pains.

Also, try to avoid devices that do not display their intensity output explicitly. Most devices that are legitimate will display the energy output or irradiance of their devices.

Tip: In considering the intensity of an RLT device, check the irradiance often represented as mW/cm2 or energy/cm2 per minute/Joules.

When the irradiance of the device is displayed, you can determine the energy intensity it can deliver to your skin using this formula: I (Irradiance) x 60 (time seconds) ÷ 1000

If, for example, the energy output of the device is given as 15 mW/cm2, the energy intensity is 15 mW/cm2 x 60/1000 = 0.9 Joules/cm2 per minute.

The example above shows that the device will not be very effective because the best devices deliver up to

4-6 Joules/cm2 per minute. Some devices offer higher intensities and deliver up to 60 Joules/cm2 to the skin. It is important to consider the intensity of the device because it controls the duration of the therapy. Therapy sessions will last longer if you use a device that is lowly powered while using a high-powered device will quickly translate into deep tissue stimulation.

2. Your lifestyle

Consider how the device you want to purchase complements your lifestyle or fits into it. How much time can you spare for at-home therapy? It is good to go for a device that delivers very high wavelengths and intensity of red light quickly and conveniently. If you cannot dedicate enough time to RLT, you should not get a small device.

Also, consider how convenient your device will be for use. First, consider the parts of your body you want to treat. For example, an RLT therapy mask is better for treating the face alone. If you want to treat your entire body, get a bigger device like a tanning bed.

3. The coverage/treatment area

Do not neglect to put the coverage area into consideration. Note that a smaller device is perfect for treating a smaller area.

The area of your skin a particular RLT device can treat or cover depends primarily on these three factors: its dimension, angle of the refracting lens, and the distance from the surface of the skin.

In terms of dimensions, there are lots of RLT LED panel devices for your particular needs. Their sizes include small, large, broad, and narrow. The type you buy depends largely on your budget. Devices with larger LED panels will cover more treatment areas, have greater energy output, and are more expensive. If it is within your budget, get a device with a bigger LED panel because it has more coverage and power density.

Therefore, know the areas you want to treat because, for example, if you want the device that treats your face, get one meant for the face alone. Do not opt for a device with one intention and then start using it in other areas.

In terms of the angle of the refracting lens, this lens is placed over the LED panel to make sure there is even the final dispersion of the red light. The lens is crucial because it ensures that emitted light is effective. Here, the majority of the manufacturers use either bare LEDs or secondary lenses.

The refracting angle of secondary lenses is 30, 60, and 90 degrees. The effect this has is that the angle of refraction will affect the coverage area. A secondary lens that has a smaller refracting angle will have a higher concentration in an area but limited coverage in other areas. A very good device will use a secondary focusing lens of a higher angle (60 degrees or more) to ensure effective coverage as well as output.

In terms of the distance between the red light and the skin surface, you should keep in mind that the farther the light is from a surface, the wider the surface area coverage. In some cases, especially where low-quality light is used, if the LED panel is farther away from the surface of the skin, there will be lowered intensity.

4. Device manufacturer and warranty

It will be a big mistake to overlook and not compare different manufacturers, their experience level, and the warranty offered.

To get value for your money, go for manufacturers with a proven record of innovation in this field and who offer a warranty they willingly stand by. The strength of a manufacturer shows the level of consumer trust. So, while thinking of which manufacturer you want to patronize, also consider the warranty period, and read reviews related to the same manufacturer to see how warranty claim processes are handled.

5. Your aim

As often mentioned, it is important to consider how you intend to use the device. If you are aiming at ensuring the light goes deeper to affect deep tissue, go for near-infrared light devices. If, on the other hand, you need RLT for skin enhancement but not treatment of arthritis or joint pains, you should use red light devices.

Large LED panels are the best for general red light therapy because of their larger coverage of 660nm to 850nm. Devices delivering a combination of these wavelengths can work for many cases like joint pains, skin condition therapy, and fat loss.

Lights of up to 660nm work best with red light for reversing hair loss and enhancing skin. If you are targeting joints, organs, as well as muscles and tendons, pure light or near-infrared devices with 850nm is ideal.

If you are concentrating on using red light therapy for enhancing the brain or as a remedy for depression, anxieties, and other psychosomatic conditions, you should use near-infrared light devices.

With these conditions in mind, while looking for RLT devices, it should be easy to narrow down your list of devices to just a few that match the way you use the red light therapy.

Red Light Therapy Dosage or Photobiomodulation

To effectively use red light therapy, you should pay close attention to the dosage. This, in most cases, means that you should pay attention to your RLT device's energy intensity at different distances away from the surface of the skin, and the duration of the therapy sessions.

The dosage of red light therapy depends on light intensity. The higher the intensity/density, the more concentrated the effect of red light at given distances. For example, some near-infrared light and red light devices have a power density of up to 450-600 MW/cm2 at a distance of 5cms from the skin or point of contact.

One fundamental thing you should note on dosage is that clinically, light devices with a density of more than 200mw/cm2 are not suitable for treating skin conditions. If, however, you use them in a controlled way and for shorter periods, these devices can be used for deep tissue stimulation like treatment of arthritis, joint pain, back pain, etc.

After determining the power density of your device, you can then determine the light therapy range, which is the distance at which to place the device. This will make sure your LED panel or red light device is placed at a distance that is appropriate for the right power density. With devices of a 10-200mW/cm2 range, the distance is often 0-35cm.

The formula

To calculate the right dosage for photobiomodulation, use this formula: Dose = Power Density x Time x 0.001

The power density is a very important consideration to be used in at-home red light therapy use. Without knowing the power density of a device, it may be difficult to calculate the ideal dosage for optimal effect.

Much high-quality near-infrared and red light devices display their light density/intensity. Some manufacturers indicate the photons in a particular area of space.

To cover a larger area, some RLT devices with such angled output LED devices take advantage of how the light spreads. In devices like this, the further light spreads out, the wider the coverage area. To compromise this, the density/intensity is weaker when it is taken further away from the base source.

The higher the light intensity or power density a device has, the less time you will need to spend under it. The majority of the benefits discussed here are from studies and clinical trials making use of lights of a power density of 10mWcm2 to 200mW/cm2.

For instance, if you intend to determine the dosage for a skin area measuring 40cm x 40cm or 1600cm2, and the red light device you want to use has 200000Mw or 200 Watts, the device may have a power density of 125mW/cm2. This is a great power density.

When you have the power density at different distances and your preferred dosage in J per cm2, you can use this formula to calculate the duration of the therapy in seconds: Time = Dose ÷ (Power density x 0.001).

Red light therapy dosage usually depends on the power density/intensity of the device, the dosage duration (the time you stay under the light), and the distance from the surface. Joules per centimeter squared (J/cm2) is the unit of measure that is used in displaying the dosage. Hence, the higher the power density, the lesser the dosage. Rather, the higher a device's power density with distance from the surface of the skin, the lower the time of application (in seconds).

Conventionally, most of the benefits of red light therapy discussed earlier become evident when the distance from the surface, which is the distance between the red light device and the skin surface, is 20mW/cm2 on the lower end and 200mW/cm2 on the higher end, especially for larger devices. When the red light therapy is placed farther away from the skin, you may have to compensate for this by increasing the treatment's duration.

The ideal dose

The ideal dosage is 3J/cm2 – 50J/cm2. However, this dosage will depend largely on why you are using red light therapy.

It is important to know that application time (how long the red light is applied to your skin at a particular distance and power density) will go a long way in influencing the damage.

More so, the effective dosage of treating acne is 5-96 J/cms2. The dosage for back pain is 40-100 J/cm2.

When considering dosage, the guideline is to get a high powered red light therapy device that will still give a larger part of your skin the appropriate light intensity for cellular activation even as you move farther away from it.

Also, the number of treatments each week will depend largely on the condition that is being treated. The general guideline for this is 2-14 treatments each week, depending on the dosage and the condition, and the best time for this red light therapy is in the mornings and evenings.

When you start with red light therapy, begin with low dosages at a very healthy distance and gradually increase the dosage while the skin surface gets accustoms to the use of red light. More so, mind that while treating areas like the highly sensitive face, you should use the dosage conservatively.

Do not forget to always use a dosage of 3J/cm2 – 50J/cm2 for general use.

To avoid overdosage that could result in negative effects when using red light therapy, more is not often better. The best thing will be to stick to the dosage range that was recommended.

Tips for Red Light Therapy

After choosing and learning how to use the right dosage to treat your condition, the next step is for you to continue to use red light therapy consistently as directed by your physician or dermatologist.

Here are some essential tips and strategies to keep in mind as you use your device to get the most out of your therapy sessions.

1. RLT can be used more than once daily

You may have more than just 1 session of red light therapy per day, we only have to keep in mind the optimal dosage and dosage's upper limit. To be clear, the appropriate dosage for this is 3Jcm2 to 50J/cm2 or even higher if you need deeper tissue stimulation.

In red light therapy as mentioned earlier, more is not better. Overdoing therapy sessions, staying too long under the light, or having too many sessions in one day, may have adverse effects on the skin, but it may not be as adverse on the skin as overdosing this on ultraviolet light, but still undesired.

The keyword is the balance in red light therapy: treatment should be a balance of using a device that has an adequate power density, placed at an ideal distance to surface/skin, and used for the right amount of time daily or weekly as advised.

In red light therapy, there is overexposure as well as underexposure. Too many sessions of red light therapy could negate any positive effect the red light therapy might have had. Underexposure, on the other hand, means no benefits whatsoever.

To enjoy the most benefits and best effects, your aim should be balanced, as optimal dosage will allow you to get as much benefit as possible from red light therapy. Most red light and near-infrared lights devices that are available and of high quality come with instructions regarding power density at different distances as well as the ideal amount of time to be taking treatment under the device (dosage) for different conditions.

The ideal dosage of RLT for a day varies depending on your goal, the power density of the device, and the time spent under the pure red light's radiance. If you do not overdo it, your RLT can then be used as many times as is deemed necessary for a day.

2. About protective gear, clothing, and makeup

The red light therapy devices that are most common are the red light facemasks or the red and near-infrared lights you may shine on different areas of your skin or farther away from your body, depending on its power density. This stirs the question of protecting the sensitive parts of the skin like the eyes by maybe wearing eye-protecting goggles or gear.

Regarding protective eye gear, a lot of researchers and experts in this field have concluded that red light therapy at a mid-600nm wavelength can have a lot of benefits to the eyes. This means that when using a device with such a red light wavelength, you don't need to use the eye-protecting gear.

If, however, you have particular light sensitivities, it is better to acclimate your eyes to red light using it in a room that is well-lit or looking at the device or away from the device in short successions. You may also shut your eyes for some seconds, open them, then look at the red light for some seconds before you close your eyes again, and then going over the process again a couple of times until your eyes become accustomed to the red light.

More so, if your device has more than mid-600nm-700nm, wear eye-protecting gear or shut your eyes during the therapy sessions to protect your eyeballs from overheating while undergoing treatment. Most of the red light or infrared red facemasks have built protective eye mechanisms internally which allow your eyes to stay open during the therapy session.

With regards to other types of protective gear like clothing, it is important to remember that in red light therapy, the more skin exposed to red light at the appropriate intensity/density and for the appropriate amount of time, the more you will benefit from the therapy.

If your red light or near-infrared device is large enough as a full-body device, you may not need to use protective gear. However, for therapy sessions, you can strip down to your undergarments. It may be necessary to wear light clothing depending on the device's density at different distances.

With regards to makeup and some beauty products like lipstick, you can still benefit from this red light therapy without taking off your 'makeup', but it is far better to clean the skin before your therapy session to get the best result. Most of these red and near-infrared light devices are of high quality come with a set of instructions. Specifically, most facemasks have a detailed procedure that indicates how to treat the skin even before and after any red light therapy session.

With regards to using the device after a bath, most available devices prefer to use high-grade electronics parts; still, they are electronics and if you want to use a red light device after either your morning or evening bath, it will be better if you first dry off.

3. Treatment guidelines

The right dosage of RLT, as mentioned earlier, depends largely on your device as well as the intended area of condition/treatment. On that note, many red lights and near-infrared light devices that are available come with a set of treatment guidelines or instructions depending on the light density of the device from different distances.

Many high quality, at-home red light devices help advocate for standing or sitting 4-6 inches away from a device because 4-6 inches away from the device is the appropriate distance from the surface which is clinically proven.

Most of the red light therapy at-home devices and treatment centers have some guidelines on how a person can get started. In some of these instances, both treatment centers and at-home devices will advocate for getting yourself into this therapy with brief sessions and increasing the duration. For example, some manufacturers recommend that people ease themselves into the therapy along with usage of the RLT device with 1-2 minutes of therapy sessions on a smaller area, then building up to sessions of 10-15 minutes in a specified time window.

Most of the treatment centers and devices will advocate for 10-15-minute sessions to ensure optimal exposure. However, the right dosage is a balance that is based on the power density at certain distances.

In the use of targeted devices, one which allows you to target a particular skin area, when you use a device like this on a particular area of the skin, like the thigh, it is better to avoid treating the area for a minimum of 6 hours. With devices that are used on the full-body, there is no need worrying about this because they shine a red light on big portions of the body, hence only require one or two therapy sessions every day. Remember that more red light may not translate to improved benefits, overexposure could negate the benefits that are intended.

Most of the at-home red light therapy devices could advocate for daily use. You can even have more than one session of therapy each day if you remember the upper limit of your dosage. If you use your device more consistently, the impact it will have on cellular activity and regeneration will be greater. Just like exercising, the benefits of red light therapy treatments increase when you create a regular treatment schedule and stick to it. More so, sticking to a schedule that is consistent and regular will ensure you get long-term benefits from the practice.

The most ideal times to use red light therapy are mornings and evenings because it is possible to schedule red light therapy into both the morning and evening routines. This will help the rejuvenation of energy in the morning, and a form of relaxing and unwinding in the evening.

The time of day you should use your red light therapy will mostly depend on the benefits you intend to accrue. For example, if you want to speed up muscle recovery after a workout, scheduling red light treatment after exercise will have the greatest effect. If, on the other hand, you want to improve sleep, it will make more sense to schedule your session of red light therapy as part of a relaxing evening or night routine. If we are asking what the appropriate time for having a red light therapy session is, the answer is you should do whatever feels appropriate for you depending on the benefits you intend to enjoy.

4. Duration to benefits

The duration of manifestation of red light therapy treatments will differ based on some factors like consistency, appropriate dosage, and many other factors like distance from the surface and the area targeted or treated.

With that in mind, intended benefits can manifest after some weeks of consistent use of RLT. In some cases like using RLT for inflammation and joint pain, some people have said they experienced red light therapy benefits after one therapy session.

For conditions like muscle and wound recovery, these benefits can manifest after 2 to 4 sessions. To treat conditions that are deeper-rooted like hair loss, joint pain, fat loss, arthritics, and so on, benefits could take some time to manifest.

The main thing to note here is that while you use the correct dosage – a red light device made of correct intensity, when kept away from the skin at the appropriate distance, with the right exposure concerning time – the benefits wanted to manifest eventually despite how long it may take.

Risk, Side Effects, and Contraindications

Generally, red light therapy is risk-free and many reputable institutions like the American Academy of Dermatology have classified it as 'safe'. Unlike UV light, pure red light has no negative effects on a person's skin. Because the therapy is also drug-free and non-invasive, it does not cause damages to the skin.

As we stated several times with RLT, more is not better. Since overexposure could have serious negative effects on the skin, remember that overdosing on RLT could negate the effects of increased ATP production and cellular activation.

In light of the above, red light therapy has some risks like when treatment in on a light-sensitive skin. For instance, the use of Accutane in the treatment of acne will increase the sensitivity of your skin to light, hence the use of red light therapy as they use Accutane could lead to skin scarring on some individuals.

Also, if you are very sensitive to sunlight or you use whatever makes you sensitive to sun rays, you will have to consult a qualified professional before you use red light therapy.

The side effects from the use of red light therapy are rare and dismal. Most clinical trials have not pointed out any serious side effects. However, minor side effects like eye strain, irritability, and headaches can happen short-term. Most of the side effects are not overtly from using red light therapy; however, they are an effect of the glare of red light, which may be intense at times.

If you acclimatize your eyes to red light as shown previously, i.e. wearing protective eye gear or closing your eyes, which is a personal decision, you could bypass the majority of these side effects. Also, you could avoid several situations that would make you stare directly into the source of red light.

As shown in some studies, when light therapy is used on individuals that were diagnosed with drug-resistant and non-seasonal depression, it tends to aggravate the situation into hyperactive mania. In such a case, the best thing to do is to consult a qualified professional and seek treatment for a condition before they embark on red light therapy.

More importantly, to avoid these side effects, it is advisable to get professional medical advice before you begin to use red light therapy.

Note: It is worth noting here that near-infrared light therapy (using red light to treat on the higher side of the spectrum of wavelength), compared to red light therapy, is more likely to have side effects. This is because near-infrared devices emit thermal energy too, and this may lead to problems like thermal burn/burning and skin overheating.

With the use of infrared light devices and therapy, try to exercise care and caution; also, be very strict with the dosage as well as the distance from the surface which depends on the power density of the distance that is in question.

Contraindication

In light of these examples, it will be great to consult before you use a red light or near-infrared light therapy:

1. Avoid using red light therapy after Botox or cosmetic filler procedure: The skin is now more sensitive and will most likely scare. Nonetheless, since red light therapy is great at healing wounds, it will be advisable to consult a physician.
2. During pregnancy: Since red light therapy is safe, as even the FDA has termed it safe for long-term use, pregnant women have to consult their physician before they use photobiomodulation.
3. Epileptic patients: If you are epileptic, it will be a good idea to consult your physician before you embark on light therapy treatments.
4. If you are suffering from Systemic Lupus Erythematosus – it is a great idea to avoid red light therapy and consult widely before you embark on using it.
5. If you have had skin-related cancers in the past, consult your physician before you use red light therapy or some other form of photobiomodulation.

The most important contraindication is that if you choose to use any medication which makes you light-sensitive, these are called photosensitizing medications; some instances include several antibiotics, melatonin, some antipsychotics, etc. – more importantly, you should avoid the use of red light or consult your physician before you use red light therapy.

Conclusion

We have examined all that should be known about red light therapy; we have discussed what it is, its benefits, how it works, how to go about the therapy, how to choose the right device and appropriate dosage, and the tips to consider concerning treatment guidelines.

Having known all these, have it in mind that red light therapy, as well as other forms of heliotherapies or photobiomodulation, are alternatives. This means that unless you are advised to do so by a professional, you should avoid anything that will cause you to use red light therapy as a great way to manage a very deep condition. As mentioned throughout this book repeatedly, it seems red light therapy works well when it is coupled with other strategies of wellbeing.

If, after you must have read this book, you decide that red light therapy has worthwhile benefits, you should consult your physician or dermatologist, then try to get a therapy session or device which will allow you expose the skin to the appropriate density of red light for the appropriate amount of time depending on the condition you want to treat.

If you follow the guidelines discussed in this guide, add that to the advice you get from a qualified physician or dermatologist, you should be capable of using red light safely and from that, get many worthwhile benefits we discussed earlier in this book.

Printed in Great Britain
by Amazon